International Medical Writing:
English for a Global Audience

clear
concise
coherent

世界に通じる メディカルライティング

ネイティブライターが伝授する 3Cs English

By **Lee Seaman** and **Tom Lang**

With contributions by **Raoul Breugelmans**, **Edward Barroga**, and **Mary Shibuya**

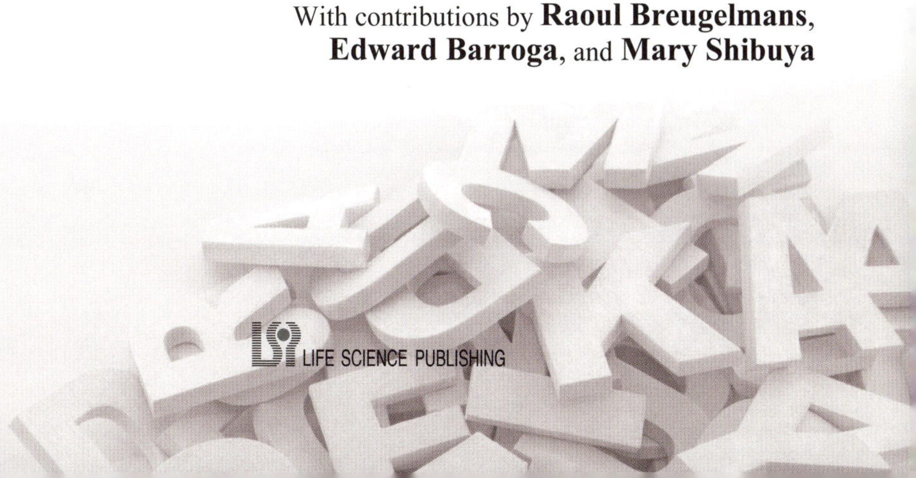

LIFE SCIENCE PUBLISHING

We are honored to dedicate this book to Professor J.Patrick Barron, the Founder and Director of the Department of International Medical Communications at Tokyo Medical University, who has probably done more than anyone to promote English-language medical writing and medical English instruction throughout Japan over the past 50 years.

Lee Seaman & Tom Lang

International Medical Writing: English for a Global Audience

ISBN 978-4-89775-388-1

First published in April 2019 by Life Science Publishing Co., Ltd.
3-5-2, Shiba, Minato-ku,Tokyo 105-0014, Japan

9 8 7 6 5 4 3 2 1

Printed in Japan
Printing / binding:Sanposya Printing Co.,Ltd.
Book Design:Ryohei Hirose

Contents

Preface はじめに

■ 3Cs English Started with Study in Japan
日本での学びに基づく 3Cs English

I began to study Japanese as a college student at Waseda University in Tokyo. There, I fell in love with the Japanese language and culture. But although most of my friends studied Japanese literature and philosophy, I studied science. I was fascinated by Japanese research, but I also found that a lot of that research was not presented well in English. As a result, most of the rest of the world did not have access to the valuable work that was being done in Japan.

After university, I studied Japanese further and began to do medical translation into English. Of course, I had to improve my Japanese, and soon I realized that my English writing skills were insufficient, too. So, I did a lot of studying, especially of medical writing, to make my translations as clear and understandable as possible.

Soon, I began to help Japanese authors with their English writing. I discovered that most of them thought in Japanese (usually complex and complicated Japanese) when they wrote in English. As a result, much of their English writing was complicated, and international readers couldn't understand it. Sometimes the authors didn't even understand their own English.

I began to teach them to write clear, simple English. Once they could understand their own writing more easily, their readers could understand it, too. That was the beginning of my thinking about 3Cs (Clear Concise Coherent) English as my goal for international medical writing. I wanted to write 3Cs English myself, and I wanted to teach that style of writing to my Japanese students.

The 3Cs relate to the text as a whole, not to vocabulary. Medical vocabulary is generally precise, clear, and widely understood by specialists around the world. As a result, we don't need to fix vocabulary. However, English grammar should be as clear and simple as possible. Fortunately, you can use several grammar techniques to make your English sentences easier to understand. In this book, Tom and I identify 12 such techniques. We call them "edits" because they are editing techniques. We think that applying these 12 edits can help you to achieve the 3Cs. We believe that this practice will help you to 1) think more clearly about what you want to say and 2) say it in a form that is more likely to be understood by your reader. The result should be writing that is clearer, more concise, and more coherent.

For example, here is a rather confusing sentence: "In the case of body mass index, it was apparent from the research that the development of insulin resistance may have been affected by it." That sentence is difficult to understand, especially for many international readers who are not native English speakers. To achieve the 3Cs, we can rewrite this sentence as "The research showed that body mass index might have affected the development of insulin resistance." This sentence is easier to understand, for the author and for both native and non-native English-speaking readers. It meets the goals of the 3Cs.

I translate and edit technical documents from Japanese to English for the pharmaceutical industry, and my co-author, Tom, edits scientific articles written by authors who are not native English speakers. We have been friends for years and recently realized that our skills in working with Japanese authors are complementary. That realization led to this book. We are grateful for the inspiration and support of our colleagues in Japan, Mary Shibuya, Edward Barroga, and Raoul Breugelmans, who contributed many hours of time and effort in reviewing drafts, suggesting edits, providing ideas, and imparting advice; to our editorial liaison, Chitose Yamaguchi, for her patience, determination, and sense of humor; and to our chief editor, Yukiko Mohri, and everyone at Life Science Publishing, for their vision in bringing this book into being.

We hope that this book will help you write more effectively, so that your international readers can understand your ideas quickly and correctly, and so that Japanese research will be more readily available to the international scientific community.

Lee Seaman
Bellingham Washington, April 2019

Introduction まえがき

■ Changes in Medical English in Japan and the World 日本と世界の医学英語の変化

In the past, language and culture barriers have made it difficult for Japanese scientists to communicate with their colleagues overseas. Japan began to participate actively in the international medical community during the Meiji period. At that time, Japanese medical researchers were primarily interested in reading English documents and learning about Western research. Much of that English-language research was written in long sentences with complex grammar. Here is a typical example, from the original version of *Gray's Anatomy*, published about 150 years ago:

> "In the construction of the human body, it would appear essential, in the first place, to provide some dense and solid texture capable of forming a framework for the support and attachment of the softer parts of the frame, and of forming cavities for the protection of the more important vital organs; and such a structure we find provided in the various bones, which form what is called the Skeleton."

When *Gray's Anatomy* was first written, medical English was expected to be difficult. Little emphasis was placed on writing that was clear and easy to understand. Japanese medical researchers learned that medical English should be complicated and that complicated sentences were better than simple sentences. This view of English made it difficult for Japanese scientists to communicate with colleagues in other countries.

The modern world is very different, and so is Japanese society. Japanese businesses are global, including many pharmaceutical companies. Today, 98% of the scientific research papers published online are in English, and about 80% of ISI* Index Journals are published in English. When you discuss your work internationally, you almost certainly use English. However, native English speakers comprise only about 5% of the world's population. Most of your readers are probably non-native English speakers like you. A large percentage of them will find English difficult.

*The Institute of Scientific Information (ISI), is a bibliographic database, founded by Eugene Garfield in 1960 and now owned by Clarivate Analytics, that introduced citation metrics into the scientific literature, especially the Impact Factor.

Many of these non-native English speakers are interested in Japanese research. However, they are busy. They do not have time to figure out unclear English. Also, most of them are probably tired. They have a lot of research to read, usually after a full day of work at their office or laboratory. Because they are busy and tired, and because English may be difficult for them, your English writing must be **clear**, **concise**, and **coherent**.

This book is designed to be short and easy to read, even on a train or bus. You can start at the Introduction, or read the 12 edits first, or go directly to the Examples and Explanations. The final section contains additional information on how to publish articles in English-language peer-reviewed journals.

Good luck on your road to writing clear, concise, coherent English!

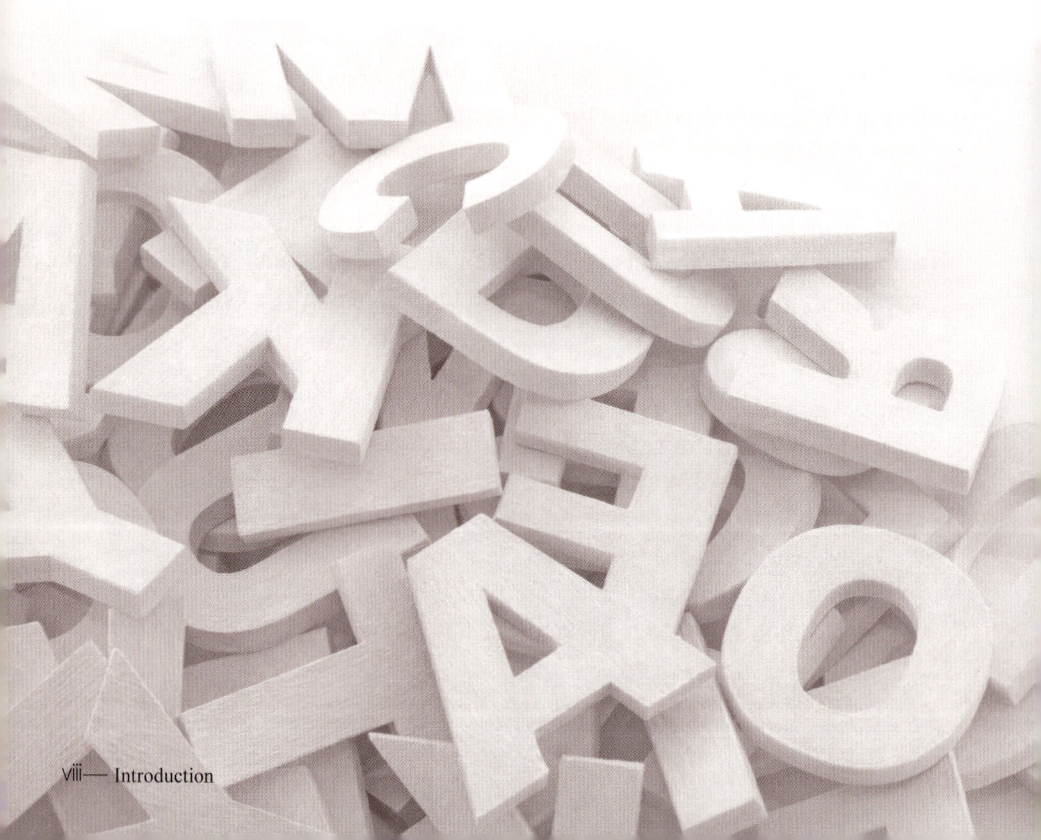

Chapter 1

Clear, Concise, and Coherent: 3Cs English

第１章　3Cs English：明快・簡潔・一貫性

ベテランのネイティブライターが辿り着いたのは，3 つの “C”。言い回しが硬くて長い文章が良い論文とは限らない。3 つの C が論文作成に有用なわけを知ろう。

Chapter 1

■ Definition of 3Cs English
3Cs Englishの極意

We suggest that the "3Cs" are pillars of effective medical writing in English for a global audience:

- The writing must be **CLEAR**.
  A reader proficient in the field should be able to understand the writing easily, without having to re-read sections or guess at the meaning. Often, you can improve reader understanding by using less-complicated grammar.

- The writing must be **CONCISE**.
  The reader does not want to read unnecessary information, such as unrelated topics, duplicate information, or unwanted details. Also, the reader wants to read quickly, and clear short sentences are faster to read than clear long ones.

- The writing must be **COHERENT**.
  All of the information must be logical, organized, complete, and related to the author's purpose.

In the Introduction, we showed the following example from *Gray's Anatomy*.

> "In the construction of the human body, it would appear essential, in the first place, to provide some dense and solid texture capable of forming a framework for the support and attachment of the softer parts of the frame, and of forming cavities for the protection of the more important vital organs; and such a structure we find provided in the various bones, which form what is called the Skeleton."

That sentence is 70 words long and is quite complicated by modern standards. The grammar is accurate and the sentence structure is correct, but today most readers do not have time for such long, complicated sentences. They need to read and understand the material quickly and accurately.

We can rewrite in clear, concise, coherent English by dividing the sentence into three sentences, like this:

> "The human body requires a framework. It must be dense and solid to support and attach to the soft tissue, and it must be capable of forming cavities to protect the vital organs. This framework is provided by the bones, which together form the skeleton."

These three sentences are 6, 27, and 12 words long, respectively, for a total of 45 words. These three sentences are about 40% shorter than the original. The grammar is much simpler, and the general meaning is easier to understand.

■ Why the 3Cs are so important in your writing
3Cs Englishが重要なわけ

First, you want to write clearly to save your readers time and effort:

- **Readers are almost always in a hurry.** If your writing is clear, concise, and coherent, your readers will be able to understand it faster and more accurately.

Second, you want to write effectively:

- **Reduce errors during writing.** After you become accustomed to applying the 12 edits of 3Cs English, you will be able to write more clearly. This clear writing will be easier to check, especially if you are checking your work against a Japanese-language source document.

- **Reduce delays because of reader misunderstanding.** Unclear English can cause readers to misunderstand the meaning. In some cases, the reader may even be too confused to ask useful questions, which can lead to frustration and delays.
- **Reduce errors during translation.** If you are translating a document from Japanese, or writing from Japanese source documents, clear, concise, coherent English will be easier to check against the Japanese. This type of English is also easier to translate into other languages, if needed.

Third, you want to be proud of your writing:

- **Good writing is good communication.** We hope that, by learning how to achieve the 3Cs, you will gain confidence and create effective and readable English medical documents.

You can apply the 12 edits that we describe in Chapter 3 to remove unnecessary words, make complicated grammar simpler and clearer, and improve reader comprehension. Each of these edits will help you to achieve the goal of all scientific writing: to help readers understand, find, remember, and use your information.

Chapter 2

Shared Experience: A Key to Improving Clarity

第２章　明快性を向上させるための鍵は，共有体験

論文を書く上で読み手の背景を認識しておくことはとても重要である。書く（話す）者と読む（聞く）者の人生体験は言わんとすることの理解に影響する。日本語で考え，それを英語化する日本人が知っておきたい世界の人々とのギャップ。

Chapter 2

■ A Culture Gap Between Japan and the World
日本と世界との間にある文化上のギャップ

Today, writers and readers often do not have much shared experience outside their professional expertise. As a writer, you need to understand how shared experience affects communication. With this understanding, you can fill in the gaps for international readers who do not share your experience. This understanding can be particularly useful if you are not accustomed to writing for readers outside Japan.

Let's look at three types of cultures: **high shared experience, moderate shared experience, and low shared experience.**

For many years, Japan has been an example of a culture with high shared experience. Today, the Japanese generation gap is widening. However, Japanese people of all ages still share many ideas and experiences in comparison to the rest of the world. The Japanese language and culture encourage ambiguity, with expressions such as 一を聞いて十を知る ("Show 1/100th of the picture, and let the student fill in the rest.") and 以心伝心 (understand each other without saying). In Japanese culture, it may actually seem insulting to "show too much" by explaining a concept completely.

Because Japan has a high level of shared experience, Japanese writers do not have to explain everything to Japanese readers. They can expect readers to fill in the gaps. They do not have to focus on writing as clearly as possible. Instead, Japanese authors often assume that their readers will "read between the lines" to understand the text.

International readers who do not share your experience may misunderstand your writing. The meaning may be ambiguous because the reader cannot fill in the missing pieces correctly. Ambiguity can have great cultural value in Japan. However, ambiguity is the opposite of the 3Cs, which are of primary importance in international medical and scientific writing. Ideally, a skilled writer will produce sentences that have only one possible meaning. You want to write so clearly that you cannot be misunderstood.

Medical writing is "reader-based" writing; writing that is focused on understanding and meeting your readers' needs for information. (In contrast, "writer-based" writing focuses on developing self-expression.) Your goal is to communicate your research to your readers. Most will be familiar with the general topic, but none know what you know about your research. You have to tell them everything they need to know because they cannot fill in any missing pieces.

Reader-based writing means that you are responsible for explaining your research to your readers as directly and as clearly as possible. You have to consider what information they want and need from you, as well as their experience. Unfortunately, the basic concepts of reader-based writing are not generally taught in high schools or universities (in Japan and most other countries). Instead, most people learn to write technical documents through on-the-job training—and from reading books like this one.

The United States is a culture with moderate shared experience. In the US, schools are controlled by local school boards and the states, rather than by the national government. Teacher qualifications, textbooks, and graduation requirements vary from one part of the country to another, and students' educational, historic, ethnic, and religious backgrounds differ more widely than they do in Japan. All these differences mean that diversity is higher—and shared experience is lower—in the US than in Japan.

Because the US and many other countries have only moderate levels of shared experience, writers cannot assume that readers will always understand them. As a result, writers have to provide more information to make sure that readers will understand the writing. In addition, most readers expect writers to write clearly, with as little ambiguity as possible.

Your international readers will probably have a lower level of shared experience than will your Japanese readers. Most of your readers will not be familiar with the Japanese language or Japanese society, and most will probably not be native English speakers.

International readers are not able to fill in many gaps because they do not share enough of your experience. So as a writer, you have to bridge those gaps. You have to communicate as directly, as specifically, and as completely as you can. You cannot assume very much, even among readers in your same field of science or medicine. You have to review your writing carefully, to make sure you have given international readers all the information they need to understand you quickly and correctly.

■ People who are doing research and people who are writing English are always busy. But international readers are busy, too.
研究者も英文執筆者も忙しい。だが，世界中の読者だって忙しい

As we said above, in many cultures, readers expect the writer to be direct and clear. A typical Japanese reader may say, “I don’t understand what the author is saying; I have to study harder.” However, an international reader will probably say, “I don’t understand what the author is saying. The author has to write more clearly and stop wasting my time or I won’t continue reading!” In medical writing, you are responsible for your readers’ understanding. It is your job to make sure that your readers can understand your document, whether they are fellow researchers, journal editors, or administrators in regulatory agencies.

Chapter 3

Writing Better in English: The 12 Edits

第３章　12の“edits”で 3Cs English をマスターしよう

3Cs English（Clear, Concise, Coherent）をマスターするための12のコツを，具体例を示しながら解説。目から鱗が落ちるぐらいの発見がある。

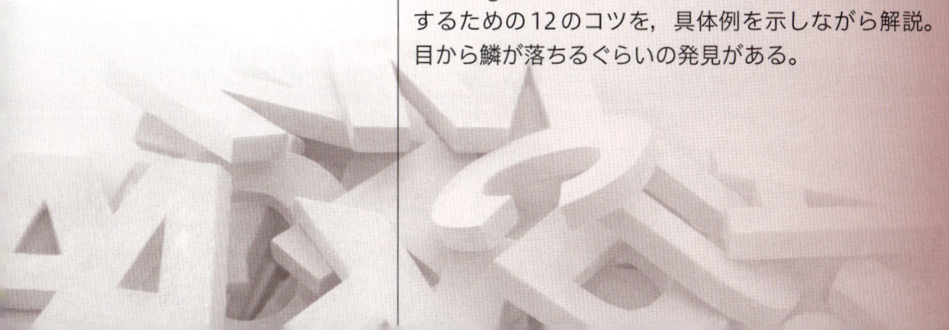

Chapter 3

We want to help you achieve the 3Cs by teaching you to fit your thoughts into sentences that use certain grammatical forms. First, you put your thoughts into English, then you edit your sentences with one or more of the 12 edits described here. These edits will help you to 1) think about what you want to say and 2) say it in a form that is more likely to be understood by your readers.

For example, a cardiologist who is quite familiar with echocardiography might write:

> Left ventricular strain is a measure of myocardial deformation and assesses myocardial function more precisely than does the longitudinal myocardial velocity gradient. This also varies with body mass index.

Here, "this" could refer to left ventricular strain, myocardial deformation, myocardial function, or the velocity gradient. Even other cardiologists may have to stop and think about the meaning.

The author could apply two of the 12 edits we describe here: use shorter sentences and ensure that the meaning of all pronouns is clear. Below, the first sentence has been divided into two sentences, and the pronoun "this" is clarified in the third sentence:

> Left ventricular strain is a measure of myocardial deformation. This measure of myocardial function is more precise than the longitudinal myocardial velocity gradient. Left ventricular strain also varies with body mass index.

Later, the author or an editor might refine these sentences into more flowing text for publication:

> Left ventricular strain is a measure of myocardial deformation, which is a more precise measure of myocardial function than the longitudinal myocardial velocity gradient. Left ventricular strain also varies with body mass index.

Here are the 12 edits that we believe will help you to write more clearly, concisely, and coherently.

1. Prefer shorter sentences.
2. Keep the verb close to the subject.
3. Avoid using empty words.
4. Prefer the active voice and "subject-verb-object" sentence structure.
5. Be careful when using the passive voice.
6. Use nominalizations only when necessary.
7. Be careful about using the passive voice and nominalizations in the same sentence.
8. Make the units of a sentence parallel when possible.
9. Use personal pronouns ("I" and "we") where appropriate.
10. Ensure that the meaning of all pronouns is clear.
11. Use only a few common standard abbreviations.
12. Use a "given-new" edit to connect your ideas and make your writing smoother.

Below, we describe these edits in detail. See Chapter 4 for more examples. To help you understand the 12 edits more easily, in each example, we have underlined the subject of the sentence once and underlined the verb twice. We have also bolded the words or phrases that are the **topic of the edit**.

1 Prefer shorter sentences.
文は短いほうが良い

Here is a long sentence that is difficult to understand:

After the completion of bench tests and studies in laboratory animals in December 2017, phase 2 studies of AB-123, which is a novel steroid-like compound, are scheduled to begin at the end of the phase 1 studies that were initiated in January 2018.

This sentence is not well organized. As you can see, the grammar is complicated and confusing. The reader cannot easily identify the subject, verb, and object of the sentence. As a result, he or she may have to read the sentence at least twice to understand it.

We can make the sentence much easier to read by breaking it into 4 short sentences. In this case, the time sequence is important, so we will organize the sentences sequentially.

- The study drug AB-123 is a new, steroid-like compound.
- Bench tests and studies of AB-123 in laboratory animals were completed in December 2017.
- Phase 1 studies were started in January 2018.
- Phase 2 studies of AB-123 are scheduled to begin after the phase 1 studies are completed.

Bullet points like these are often used in PowerPoint presentations. However, journal articles and regulatory documents contain far more paragraphs than bulleted lists. We can convert these bullet points into a paragraph by rewriting them slightly. The resulting three sentences are easy to read and understand:

The study drug AB-123 is a new steroid-like compound. Bench tests and studies in laboratory animals were completed in December 2017, and phase 1 studies were started in January 2018. Phase 2 studies of the drug are scheduled to begin after the phase 1 studies are completed.

Complicated grammar is often confusing, and confusion is the enemy of quick and correct understanding. You should thus avoid complicated grammar as much as possible. Shorter sentences are less likely to be complicated, so we generally recommend sentences of 20 words or less, especially for your first draft. Of course this is only a guideline; you should use more than 20 words if needed. Do try to keep the grammar simple, however.

In your second draft, you can combine some short sentences to make longer sentences that are equally understandable. In the example above, the middle sentence was created by combining two sentences: "Bench tests and studies in laboratory animals were completed in December 2017." and "Phase 1 studies were begun in January 2018."

Long sentences do not have to be confusing; if the grammar is not complicated, even long sentences can be easy to read. At the end of this chapter, we show you how to use parallel structure to create longer sentences that are still easy to read.

However, clear, well-organized, short sentences are generally easier to write than clear, well-organized long sentences. We thus encourage you to write short sentences, especially while you are learning to achieve 3Cs English.

2 Keep the verb close to the subject.
動詞は主語の近くに置く

The reader can usually understand the sentence better if the subject and verb are close together. In this example, the subject and verb are separated by 20 words.

Every step of the procedure, including the criteria for selecting patients, the surgical approach, the operative technique, and the postoperative nursing care, had to be evaluated.

Here, the author has introduced a lot of information after the subject. But where is the verb? Readers have to search for it. At the same time, they also have to keep the subject and the other information in short-term memory. Finding the verb can be hard work, especially if English is not the reader's native language. We can reorganize the sentence like this:

Every step of the procedure had to be evaluated, including the criteria for selecting patients, the surgical approach, the operative technique, and the postoperative nursing care.

3 Avoid using empty words.
無意味な言葉は使わない

"Empty" words do not add any meaning to the sentence, and they require extra time to read. We want readers to understand the information quickly and correctly, so we should remove empty words and phrases wherever possible. This sentence contains empty words:

In April 2015, the regulatory authorities **issued an announcement, which introduced** a proposed regulatory framework for immunotherapy products.

The words "issued an announcement, which introduced" do not add any information. We can delete them, and the sentence will be shorter and easier to read.

In April 2015, the regulatory authorities proposed a regulatory framework for immunotherapy products.

The phrases "there is," "there are," "it is," and "it was" do not contain information. These words are sometimes helpful for grammatical reasons, but they should not be overused. In particular, they are often found with the words "that" or "which." If they add no information, these phrases can usually be removed. Here are some examples.

With empty words (in bold)	Without empty words
There are many ways in which the surgery can be done.	The surgery can be done in many ways.
It was thought that transfusions were dangerous.	Transfusions were thought to be dangerous.
To determine whether **there are** loci that are associated with SAD status, we performed genome-wide mediation modeling.	To determine whether loci are associated with SAD status, we performed genome-wide mediation modeling.
There were five patients in each group **that** required treatment.	Five patients in each group required treatment.
The incidence of cardiovascular disease in women is lower than **it is** in men.	The incidence of cardiovascular disease in women is lower than in men.

4 Prefer the active voice and "subject-verb-object" sentence structure.

できるだけ，能動態と「主語＋述語＋目的語」の構文を用いる

In English, verbs that express action are called "action" verbs. Sentences with action verbs are said to be in the "active voice" because the subject performs that action on the object. The pattern is "[subject] [verb] [object]"; for example, "The nurse [subject] examined [verb] the stitches [object]."

Here are some examples of sentences in the active voice. Please see the next section for more information about the passive voice. The object of the sentences is in bold.

The doctor sedated the **patient**.

The laboratory technician calibrated the **scales** daily.

The sponsor and the clinic administrator signed the **contract** on March 1.

The *AMA Manual of Style* states that "In general, authors should use the active voice, except in instances in which the author is unknown or the interest focuses on what is acted upon." The subject-verb-object sentence is generally easier to read and is relatively easy to write correctly.

5 Be careful when using the passive voice.

受動態を使う時は，慎重に

Another class of verbs in English express "state-of-being." They are forms of the verb "to be": is, are, am, was, were, has been, have been, had been, will be, will have been, and being. Sentences that use one of these forms of the verb "to be" often also include other verbs ending with "-ed." This

combination is the passive voice, in which the object of the sentence is placed in the subject position. Instead of "The drug reduced the **symptoms**," the sentence becomes "The symptoms were reduced by the drug." "Symptoms" is now the subject, and "were reduced" is the verb.
To emphasize the "who" or "what" of an action, the active voice is fine. However, in some situations, "who" or "what" is not important, and the passive voice may be more appropriate.

The passive voice is useful in two situations:

a) When we do not know who or what caused the action. In the sentence, "We know that mistakes were made," the authors do not know who made the mistakes. (The authors may also not want to say who made the mistakes. In fact, the passive voice is often used to avoid assigning responsibility for an action.)

b) When what was done is more important than who did it. For example, the sentence "The rats were killed by lethal injection on March 1," has two important points: 1) the rats were killed on March 1, and 2) the rats were killed by lethal injection. In most cases, we do not need to know who killed the rats. With the passive voice, we can focus on what was done rather than on who did it.

Especially in the Methods section of papers and regulatory materials, the passive voice is often appropriate because information about "who" is not necessary. For example, the sentence, "The patients submitted their signed informed consent **forms** to the study staff" is in the active voice. However, the fact that the forms were submitted is more important than repeating the obvious fact that patients submitted them. Thus, the passive voice may be preferred, "Signed informed consent **forms** were submitted to the study staff."

Here are some other examples in which the passive voice (the right side of the box) may be better than the active voice:

Active voice	**Passive voice**
The laboratory technician calibrated the **scales** daily.	The scales were calibrated daily.
The sponsor and the clinic administrator signed the **contract** in March.	The contract was signed in March.
The doctor sedated the **patient**.	The patient was sedated.

The passive voice was once widely used in medical and scientific writing because it was thought to be more objective. However, today most medical and scientific style manuals encourage the active voice.

6 Use nominalizations only when necessary.
名詞化はどうしても必要な時にだけ

A nominalization is a verb (and sometimes an adjective) that has been turned into a noun. When a sentence loses a verb because it has been nominalized, a new verb has to be added to make the sentence complete. Usually, the replacement verb is less specific and weaker than the nominalized one, which weakens the sentence.

For example, the verb "reverse" ("The current reverses every 0.02 seconds") can be nominalized to the noun "reversal" ("Current reversal occurs every 0.02 seconds"). Here, the replacement verb "occurs" is less specific than the original verb, "reverses." In general, sentences with nominalizations are more difficult to understand.

In the examples below, notice that the nominalization may also be the subject or object of the sentence. Sometimes, you have to look carefully to find the nominalized verb, shown in bold below.

With a nominalization (in bold)	With the active verb
The technicians implemented data **collection** from 12:00.	The technicians collected data from 12:00.
Application of the ointment was performed twice daily.	The ointment was applied twice daily.
Statisticians will conduct an **analysis** of the data after the database is locked.	Statisticians will analyze the data after the database is locked.

Unfortunately, the use of nominalizations tends to lead to more nominalizations in the same sentence. For example, this sentence has two nominalizations ("confusion" and "failure"):

The **confusion** of the intern caused her **failure** on the test.

This sentence is not long, but most readers cannot understand it easily. If we remove the nominalizations, the sentence is easier to read:

The intern was confused and failed the test.

Also, unfortunately, nominalizations are often accompanied by prepositional phrases. In addition to making the sentence longer and more complex, such prepositional phrases often contain other nominalizations. However, not all nominalizations weaken the sentence; sometimes, they work better as nouns than as verbs. Examples include an operation (to operate), a response (to respond), a thought (to think), satisfaction (to satisfy), and an examination (to examine). With practice, you will learn which nominalizations weaken a sentence and which do not.

This sentence has four prepositional phrases [in brackets] and three nominalizations:

The **reduction** [in patient **satisfaction**] was caused [by the lack] [of a favorable **response**] [among physicians].

This sentence will be stronger and clearer if we change the nominalization "reduction" to the active verb "reduced." This change also removes two of the prepositional phrases:

The lack [of a favorable **response**] [among physicians] reduced patient **satisfaction**.

We can even eliminate the nominalization "response" and the remaining prepositional phrases.

The physicians did not respond favorably, which reduced patient **satisfaction**.

"Satisfaction" although still a nominalization, works well in this sentence.

Nominalizations can often be identified by the presence of weak, generic verbs:

With the nominalization (in bold)	Without the nominalization
Samples of the solution were taken for testing.	We sampled the solution for testing.
They made the **decision** to continue.	They decided to continue.
The surgeon performed the **operation** at 10 am.	The surgeon operated at 10 am.

Nominalizations can also be identified by the presence of several prepositional phrases:

> The **organization** [of the **training**] was performed [by the physicians and nurses].
> ➡ The physicians and nurses organized the **training**.

(Here, "training" is a nominalization of "to train" but again, it does not weaken the sentence.)

Finally, nominalizations can be identified by certain word endings:

organizaTION ➡ organize	productivITY ➡ productive
assignMENT ➡ assigned	preparedNESS ➡ prepare
decisION ➡ decide	organizaTION ➡ organize
removAL ➡ remove	assistANCE ➡ assist

7 Be careful about using the passive voice and nominalizations in the same sentence.

受動態と名詞化を同じ文中で使う時は，くれぐれも慎重に

The passive voice can be especially difficult to understand when it is combined with nominalizations in the same sentence. Here are some examples. As you can see, in these examples the nominalization is also the subject. In the first example, the nominalization "inspiration" works well as a noun and does not weaken the sentence.

Passive voice with a nominalization	Passive voice without the nominalization	Active voice without the nominalization
Flow **reversal** is noted during inspiration.	Flow is reversed during inspiration.	Flow reverses during inspiration.
Regeneration of the resin bed was achieved by a calcium chloride solution.	The resin bed was regenerated by a calcium chloride solution.	A calcium chloride solution regenerated the resin bed.
Expectations that the committee will reach a decision on that issue have been expressed.	The committee is expected to decide that issue.	The committee expects to decide that issue.

8 Make the units of a sentence parallel when possible.
可能であれば，パラレル構造にしよう

To make writing coherent, we can use organizational tools such as parallel structure. In parallel structure, we use a pattern to show that two or more items are similar in content or function. We do this by repeating a grammatical form in the sentence. This repetition will help the reader to understand the relationships among ideas. You can learn to use parallel structure by making lists.

Here is a simple list:

The pharmaceutical company

a. manufactured a cancer drug

b. had been manufacturing a drug for lowering lipid concentrations

c. was also a manufacturer of an immunosuppressant

This list is not parallel. If we look at the verbs, for example, we see “manufactured” in “a” and “had been manufacturing” in “b,” and in “c” the verb has become a noun, “manufacturer.”

We can create parallel structure in this simple list as follows:

The pharmaceutical company

a. manufactured a cancer drug

b. manufactured a lipid-lowering drug

c. manufactured an immunosuppressant

Now the verbs are the same, so we can rewrite the list like this:

The pharmaceutical company manufactured

a. a cancer drug

b. a lipid-lowering drug

c. an immunosuppressant

Now we can create a very simple sentence from this list:

> The pharmaceutical company manufactured **a cancer drug, a lipid-lowering drug**, and **an immunosuppressant**.

Here is a slightly more complex list with parallel structure:

> The pharmaceutical company manufactured
>
> a. a cancer drug based on cisplatin
>
> b. a lipid-lowering drug related to atorvastatin
>
> c. an immunosuppressant similar to cyclosporine

The resulting sentence is a little longer than our goal of 20 words or less, but it is easy to understand because of the parallel structure:

> The pharmaceutical company manufactured **a cancer drug** based on cisplatin, **a lipid-lowering drug** related to atorvastatin, and **an immunosuppressant** similar to cyclosporine.

The parallel structure organizes the information and makes it easier understanding. Even long sentences can be relatively easy to read if they have good parallel structure.

Here are some additional examples of parallel structure. As you can see, sometimes a parallel structure can reduce the length of sentences. The parallel parts are in **bold**.

Without parallel structure	With parallel structure
The surgeon prefers the fascia to be dissected, excising the tumor, and wide margins. [14 words]	The surgeon prefers to **dissect** the fascia, **excise** the tumor, and **leave** wide margins. [14 words]
Boys have been shown to have a higher risk of having a coronary artery lesion compared with girls. [16 words]	The risk of a coronary artery lesion was higher **in boys** than **in girls**. [14 words; 13% shorter]
In addition, 24 respondents (31%) thought that anti-tobacco campaigns were effective in smoking cessation, there were 23 respondents (30%) who preferred advertisements on TV, and health-warning labels on cigarette packaging were selected by 21 respondents (27.3%). [37 words]	When we asked respondents to identify effective strategies to reduce smoking, **24 chose** anti-tobacco campaigns, **23 chose** television advertisements, and **21 chose** health-warning labels on cigarette packaging. [27 words; 27% shorter]

9 Use personal pronouns ("I" and "we") where appropriate.

「私」とか「私たち」のような人称代名詞を効果的に使う

The personal pronouns "I," "me," "you," "we," and "us" have been acceptable in medical writing for almost 100 years. Personal pronouns make the meaning more direct and help avoid the passive voice. For example, "We completed the research in 3 months" is more direct than "The authors completed the research in 3 months." "I determined that higher doses were more effective" is more direct than "The author determined that higher doses were more effective."

Another example, "It is believed that closing a wound with hand sutures is less expensive than stapling." This sentence is in the passive voice, and the meaning of the pronoun "it" is unclear. We can rewrite the sentence more clearly by using the personal pronoun: "We believe that closing a wound with hand sutures is less expensive than stapling."

10 Ensure that the meaning of pronouns is clear.
代名詞の中味が明確であるかどうかを確認する

The pronouns, "he," "she," "it," "them," and "they," refer to a noun earlier in the text. However, if other nouns separate the pronoun and its noun, the meaning may not be clear. For example, in the sentence, "[You] Place the test tube in the hot water bath, adjust the thermostat, and shake **it** occasionally," what does "it" refer to? What is being shaken: the test tube or the thermostat? We can rewrite this sentence as "[You] Place the **test tube** in the hot water bath, adjust the thermostat, and shake the **test tube** occasionally."

"That" and "which" are also sometimes used as pronouns: "Pick that up"; "The cells, which were infected, were harvested for further study."

As your writing improves, you may begin to see that the meaning of these and other pronouns may not be clear: any, anything, each, no one, someone, everybody, both, several, and many; there are many others.

11 Use only a few common standard abbreviations.
略語は一般的で標準的なものだけを使う

Abbreviations can be useful, but only if their meaning is known or can be found and remembered easily. Many readers find abbreviations difficult to remember. Thus, use abbreviations only if they are listed in standard reference manuals, reduce the word count, and are used often in the document. Avoid abbreviations of single words, such as US for "ultrasound" or OS for "osteosarcoma." Such abbreviations do not reduce the word count but still have to be remembered to understand the text.

Define all abbreviations at first mention. Undefined abbreviations are often not understood, especially if they are unfamiliar to the readers. In addition, some abbreviations can have several plausible meanings. For example, UA can mean ultrasonic arteriography, unstable angina, upper airway, or urinary albumin.

Use only a few abbreviations. Even if they are familiar, too many abbreviations in a sentence can be difficult to read, for example: "The NHLBI-funded CHAART study of HEU children found that in utero exposure to ARVs was associated with changes in LVEF, LV contractility, and ST/PW ratio at age 2 years."

ALWAYS spell out abbreviations on first use in the body text and in the abstract. Never assume that your reader will know what an abbreviation stands for, even if it is familiar to you. For example, here are 16 more meanings for the abbreviation UA found in medical texts:

ulnar artery	ursolic acid	umbilical artery
unattended	undifferentiated arthritis	unmeasured anions
unicystic ameloblastoma	unit administer	upper arm
uranyl acetate	uric acid	urinalysis
urine aldosterone	uterine activity	uterine artery
uterine aspiration		

There are also numerous "look-alike" abbreviation such as μA (microampere) and U/A (upon arrival).

12 Use a "given-new" edit to connect your ideas and make your writing smoother.

文をつなげたり滑らかにするために,「given-new」編集を試みる

With a given-new edit, "new" information (usually at the end of the sentence) is tied to "given" or known information (usually at the beginning of the sentence). This relationship is marked by "echo words." These echo words tie sentences together by making the transitions between them easier, which improves the flow of the writing. Below is a sentence without "echo words."

The hospital installed its new computer system in 2015 and upgraded it in 2018 to accommodate the new diagnostic categories. This presented medical staff with new reporting problems, which is why we scheduled today's meeting.

We can rewrite with shorter sentences and "echo words," as shown below. The echo words are in **bold**.

The hospital installed its new computer **system** in 2015. The **system** was upgraded in 2018 to accommodate the **new diagnostic categories**. The **system** and the **new categories** have presented medical staff with **new reporting problems**. These **problems** are the subject of today's meeting.

We'll look at more examples of how to apply these 12 edits in the next chapter.

Chapter 4

Examples and Explanations

第 4 章　例文解説

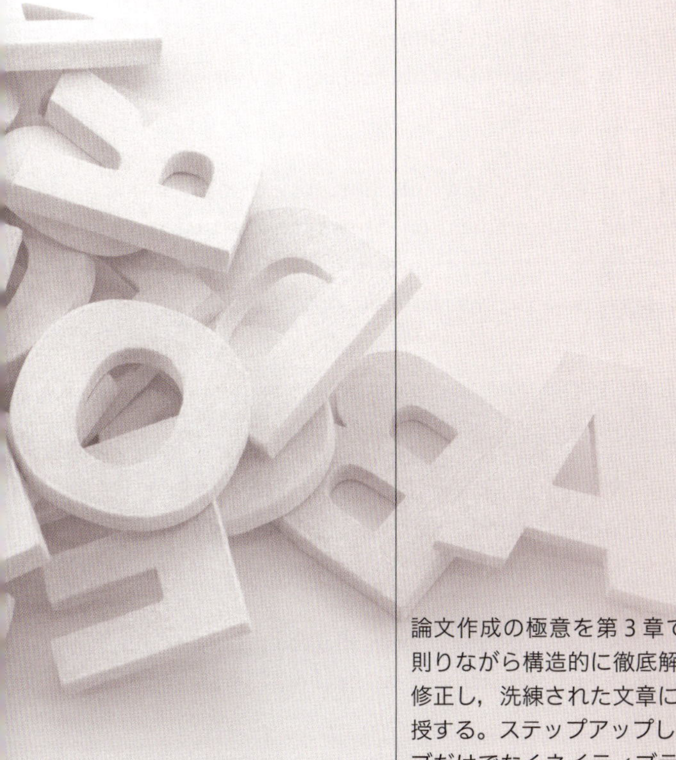

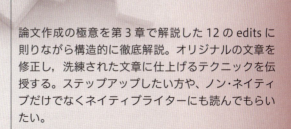

論文作成の極意を第 3 章で解説した 12 の edits に則りながら構造的に徹底解説。オリジナルの文章を修正し，洗練された文章に仕上げるテクニックを伝授する。ステップアップしたい方や、ノン・ネイティブだけでなくネイティブライターにも読んでもらいたい。

Chapter 4

Edit 1: Prefer shorter sentences.

1.

Original sentence: Although one of the few inflammatory conditions that can be completely controlled by appropriate medication, data from an insurance database show that gout is often undertreated, perhaps because of concerns about the risk of eliciting a gout attack. [38 words]

Revised sentence: Gout is one of the few inflammatory disorders that can be completely controlled by appropriate medication. However, the disease is often undertreated, according to data from an insurance database. This may be due to concerns about the risk of eliciting a gout attack. [The three sentences in the revision are 16, 13, and 14 words, respectively, or 43 words total.]

Refined sentence: Gout is one of the few inflammatory disorders that can be completely controlled with medication. However, the disease is often undertreated, according to data from an insurance database[1]. This undertreatment[2] may be related[3] to concerns about the risk of causing a gout attack.

Commentary

▼

1. The phrase, "data from an insurance database" is too vague to be useful. Either the database needs to be identified or, better, a reference should be provided to support the claim.

2. "Undertreatment" has been added to clarify that the pronoun "this" refers to undertreatment. "Undertreatment" also echoes "undertreated" in the previous sentence.

3. The phrase, "due to," should be used only in the sense of meeting a deadline (eg, "The grant was due to the agency by 5 pm.") Otherwise,

"due to" should be replaced with "a response to," "because of," "as a result of," "related to," or "owing to."

2.

Original sentence: As for the fact that a high percentage of hyperlipidemic patients are treated with low-dose statin therapy, possibly due in part to recent discussions in the news of a potential correlation between high-dose statin therapy and stroke, it is suggested that many Japanese physicians are concerned with cerebrovascular risk in comparison to cardiovascular risk. [54 words]

Revised sentence: A high percentage of hyperlipidemic patients in Japan are treated with low-dose statin therapy. This may be due in part to recent discussions in the news about a possible correlation between high-dose statin therapy and stroke. Such findings suggest that many Japanese physicians are more concerned with cerebrovascular risk than with cardiovascular risk. [14+22+17=53 words]

Refined sentence: Large numbers[1] of patients with hyperlipidemia in Japan are treated with low-dose statin therapy. The extensive use of this therapy[2] may be a response to[3] recent discussions about a possible association between high-dose statin therapy and stroke. Such a response[4] suggests that many Japanese physicians are more concerned with the risk of stroke than with the risk of heart attack. [14+23+23=60 words]

Commentary

▼

1. In the original sentence, the subject of the author's thought is really "percentage," although the grammatical subject of the sentence is "it." "Percentage" requires a singular verb, "is." The combination of "patients . . . are" is often accepted, but it is awkward. Rewriting to "numbers . . . are" avoids the problem.

2. In the original, "this" is unclear. In fact, "this" refers to "the extensive use of statin therapy," as indicated in the revised sentence. "Therapy" in the first sentence is echoed here.

3. Here, "a response to" replaces "due to," for the reasons given in the first example.

4. "Response" is an echo word from the previous sentence.

Edit 2: Keep the verb close to the subject.

1.

Original sentence: Subjects who had completed the first segment of the study were eligible to participate in the second segment.

Revised sentence: Subjects were eligible to participate in the second segment of the study after they completed the first segment.

Refined sentence: Subjects were eligible[1] to participate in the second segment of the study after completing the first[2].

Commentary

▼

1. Both the revised and refined sentences moved the verb closer to the subject with good effect.

2. The refined sentence eliminates "they" and "segment" because they are not needed to understand the sentence correctly.

2.

Original sentence: The investigator, a cardiovascular surgeon who was conducting a study on the effects of hypercholesterolemia, planned and implemented an Internet survey as part of his study. [26 words]

Revised sentence: The investigator was a cardiovascular surgeon who was conducting a study on the effects of hypercholesterolemia. He planned and implemented an Internet survey as part of his study. [16+12=28 words]

Refined sentence: The investigator, a cardiovascular surgeon, planned and implemented an Internet survey as part of a study on the effects of hypercholesterolemia. [21 words]

> **Commentary ▶** The revised sentence is 28 words long, and the refined sentence is 21, 25% shorter. The refined sentence eliminates the duplicated meaning of pronouns "who," "he," and "his" and the phrase, "as part of his study."

Edit 3: Avoid using empty words.

Below, the empty words are in **bold**.

1.

Original sentence: It appears that the study data have been reported incorrectly.

Revised sentence: The study data appear to have been reported incorrectly.

> **Commentary ▶** The revised sentence replaces "it appears" with the more specific subject and verb, "data appear." This replacement allows "that" to be eliminated. The form of the original sentence is common and undesirable; the revised sentence is the usual revision. (Remember that "data"is plural.The singular"datun"is rarely used:"data are,"not "data is.")

2.

Original sentence: We measured whether **there were** differences in BMD between study start and study end.

Revised sentence: We measured differences in BMD between study start and study end.

Refined sentence: We measured the change[1] in bone mineral density[2] between the beginning and end of the study.[3]

Commentary

▼

1. The revised sentence replaces "whether there were" with "differences" as the object of the sentence. The refined sentence replaced "differences" with "change" because it is singular (ie, "differences" means more than one) and because it indicates what the authors are interested in: the change in a variable, not just the differences between two measurements.

2. The abbreviation BMD should be spelled out, unless it is used commonly in the full text and is defined at first mention.

3."Between study start and study end" reads like a note in a laboratory notebook. "Between the beginning and end of the study" is standard English.

Edit 4: Prefer the active voice and "subject-verb-object" sentence structure.

Below, the objects (active voice) / subjects (passive voice) are in **bold.**

1.

Original sentence: The consent **form** was signed by the patient.

Revised sentence: The patient[1] signed[2] the consent **form**.

Commentary

▼

1. The passive voice uses a form of the verb "to be" (here, "was signed") and uses the intended object of the sentence ("form," in **bold**) as the subject of the sentence.

2. The active voice identifies who did what action: "patient signed."

2.

Original sentence: The **results** of the laboratory analysis, which the client conducted at a central testing facility, were entered by hospital staff into each patient's chart.

Revised sentence: The client conducted laboratory **analyzed** at a central testing facility, and hospital staff entered the **results** into each patient's chart.

Refined sentence: The results were determined[1,2] at a central testing laboratory[3] and entered into patient's charts by hospital staff[4].

Commentary

▼

1. Although the revised sentence is in the active voice, the topic of the thought is "results." The fact that the results were "determined and

entered" is more important than knowing who determined and entered them, making the passive voice appropriate in the refined sentence.

2. Both the original and revised sentences use the nominalization "analysis," which requires adding the generic verb with little meaning, "conducted."

3. "Laboratory," a more specific noun, replaces "facility," a less-specific noun.

4. The changes reduced the length of the sentence by 29%, from 24 words to 17.

Edit 5: Be careful when using the passive voice.

Below, the objects (active voice) / subjects (passive voice) are in **bold.**

1. Passive voice preferred

Original sentence: The staff cleaned and tested the **machines** every morning before the start of production.

Revised sentence: The **machines** were cleaned and tested every morning before the start of production.

Commentary ▶ The revised sentence does what needs to be done: it focuses attention on the fact that the machines were cleaned and tested and away from the obvious fact that someone (staff) cleaned and tested them.

2. Passive voice not preferred

Original sentence: Medical emergency **calls** will be answered by someone 24 hours a day.

Revised sentence: Someone will answer medical emergency **calls** 24 hours a day.

Refined sentence: The on-call physician will answer medical emergency **calls** 24 hours a day.

Commentary ▶ The original sentence indicates that "calls will be answered," which may be appropriate, depending on the context, assuming that we don't care who "someone" is. The revised sentence adds no information; obviously, phones are answered by "someone." The refined sentence assumes we will want or need to know that the calls will be answered by a physician qualified to give advice in emergencies. If so, the active voice calls attention to this fact.

Edit 6. Use nominalizations only when necessary.

Below, the nominalizations and related verbs are in **bold.**

1.

Original sentence: The nurse will handle **sterilization** of the surgical field.

Revised sentence: The nurse **will sterilize** the surgical field.

Commentary ▶ The problem with nominalizations is that many are accepted nouns that can and should be used as nouns or adjectives, whereas others are better used as verbs. Here, for example, "sterile" is useful as an adjective (a sterile procedure), and "sterilization" is useful as a noun (sterilization is more expensive than disinfection). In the example, "will handle" is a weaker verb than "will sterilize," so the nominalization should be converted back to the active verb.

2.

Original sentence: A **retraction** of the paper was issued by the journal at the request of the corresponding author.

Revised sentence: The journal **retracted** the paper at the request of the corresponding author.

> **Commentary ▶** Turning "retracted" into the normalization, "retraction," required adding a weaker verb, "was issued," to the sentence and changing the sentence from the active to the passive voice.

Edit 7: Be careful about using the passive voice and nominalizations in the same sentence.

Below, the nominalizations and related verbs are in **bold.**

1.

Original sentence: The **evaluation** of the clinical study was conducted by the academic investigators, without input from the sponsor.

Revised sentence: The academic investigators **evaluated** the clinical study, without input from the sponsor.

> **Commentary ▶** Sentences in the passive voice with nominalizations are difficult to understand because the true subject and verb are hard to identify. Unfortunately, nominalizations also encourage the use of the passive voice, so this combination is common.

2.

Original sentence: The **inability** to read the small print on the pill bottle was responsible for several dosing errors among the elderly patients. [21 words]

Revised sentence: Some elderly patients were **unable** to read the small print on their pill bottles. This small print was responsible for several dosing errors. [23 words]

Refined sentence: Elderly patients **unable** to read the small print on their pill bottles made several dosing errors. [16 words]

> **Commentary ▶** Dividing the original sentence into two sentences makes the meaning clearer, but both sentences contain unnecessary words. The refined sentence is 16 words, 24% shorter than the original one at 21 words.

Edit 8: Make the units of a sentence parallel when possible.

Below, the parallel units are in **bold**.

1.

Original sentence: In addition to blood samples at each visit to the study center, it was decided that staff would collect urine samples at visits 4 and 8 and that sputum samples will be obtained at visits 4 and 12. [38 words]

Revised sentence: Staff will collect **blood samples** at each visit to the study center, **urine samples** at visits 4 and 8, and **sputum samples** at visits 4 and 12. [27 words]

> **Commentary ▶** The revised sentence does not include the 4 empty words and has only one verb (will collect), not three (was decided, will collect, and will be obtained), which eliminates 5 more words. Removing "in addition to" eliminates 3 more words. Overall, the revised sentence has 27 words and is 11 words (29%) shorter than the original, at 38 words.

2.

Original sentence: Research was conducted to determine whether AB-123 was safe and effective and whether it was well-tolerated for long-term administration.

Revised sentence: AB-123 was assessed for **safety**, **effectiveness**, and long-term **tolerability**.

> **Commentary ▶** The terms used for each of the three characteristics change form in the revised sentence. The changes in word forms needed to make a parallel structure are not always easy to recognize.

Edit 9: Use personal pronouns ("I" and "we") where appropriate.

Below, the personal pronouns are in **bold**. Pronouns that are "an understood subject" are in [**brackets**].

1.

Original sentence: The patients were asked to contact the call center immediately if they experienced any gastrointestinal pain or nausea.

Revised sentence: **We** asked the patients to contact the call center immediately if they experienced any gastrointestinal pain or nausea.

Refined sentence: **We** asked patients to contact **us** immediately if they were having gastrointestinal pain or nausea.

> **Commentary ▶** The most common personal pronouns in medical writing are I, we, and us. Personal pronouns have been acceptable in medical writing for more than 100 years. Text without personal pronouns is not "more objective" than text with them, although this

argument is still occasionally made. The words,"were having"are simpler and thus easier to understand than"experienced."

2.

Original sentence: In this chapter, the authors summarize their research on synthetic cruciate ligaments. Readers interested in synthetic menisci should see Chapter 17.

Revised sentence: In this chapter, **we** summarize our research on synthetic cruciate ligaments. For **our** research on synthetic menisci, [**you**] see Chapter 17.

> **Commentary ▶** Personal pronouns are often found in introductions and discussions, where authors talk about their work. Although difficult to see, the subject of the revised sentence is the personal pronoun, "you," which is "an understood subject."

Edit 10: Ensure that the meaning of all pronouns is clear.

Below, the pronouns of interest are in **bold**.

1.

Original sentence: The intern asked the doctor whether **she** was correct.

Revised sentence: The intern asked the doctor whether the doctor was correct. Or: The intern wanted to know whether **she** was correct and so asked the doctor.

Refined sentence: The intern asked the doctor whether **she**, the intern, was correct.

Commentary
▼

1. Assuming that both the intern and the doctor are women, the pronouns "she" and "her" could refer to either woman. Thus, in the original sentence, we don't know which one was asked about being correct.

2. The revised sentences are awkward and wordy.

3. The refined sentence solves the problem by identifying "she" as the intern by setting off "the intern" with commas.

2.

Original sentence: **It** says on the label that this medicine has mild side effects.

Revised sentence: The label states that this medicine has mild side effects.

Commentary ▶ In the original sentence, "it," although the subject of the sentence, doesn't refer to anything. The revised sentence makes clear that the label was "saying" or "states" by putting it in the subject position.

Edit 11: Use only a few common standard abbreviations.

1. The same abbreviation can have different meanings in different contexts

Original sentence: Tom was proud to have published an article in *JAMA*.

Revised sentence: Tom was proud to have published an article in the *Journal of Asian Martial Arts*.

> **Commentary ▶** Even common abbreviations may have different meanings in a different context.

2. Do not use too many abbreviations

Original sentence: 75 yo M BIBEMS c h/o CAD (s/p 3v CABG), HTN, DM2, p/w SOB x 1d.

Translated sentence: 75-year-old male brought in by emergency medical services, with a history of coronary artery disease (has had a 3-vessel coronary artery bypass graft), hypertension, diabetes, presents with shortness of breath for 1 day.

> **Commentary ▶** Self-explanatory. Using too many abbreviations turns text into a code that makes reading difficult even for people who know the code.

Edit 12: Use the "given-new" edit to connect your ideas and make your writing smoother.

Given and new words are in **bold**.

1.

Original sentence: Type 2 diabetes is increasing around the world, due at least in part to easy access to highly refined carbohydrates in the form of snack foods, which tend to be relatively inexpensive as well as extremely tasty.

Revised sentence: Type 2 diabetes is increasing around the world. This is due at least in part to easy access to highly refined carbohydrates in the form of **snack foods**. Such **foods** tend to be relatively inexpensive as well as extremely tasty.

Refined sentence: The incidence[1] of Type 2 diabetes is **increasing** around the world. This **increase**[2] is caused,[3] at least in part, by easy access to highly refined carbohydrates in the form of **snack foods**. Such **foods**[4] tend to be relatively inexpensive as well as tasty.

Commentary

▼

1. The expression "type 2 diabetes is increasing" is often seen in the popular press. However, "the incidence of type 2 diabetes" is more accurate and is a better choice for academic journals.

2. "Increase" is an echo word from the first sentence ("increasing") that helps maintain continuity between sentences.

3. As discussed above in the first edit, the phrase, "due to," is reserved for "meeting a deadline" ("The grant was due to the agency by 5 pm.") Otherwise, "due to" should be replaced with phrases such as "is caused," "because of," "as a result of," "related to," or "owing to."

4. "Foods" is another echo word.

2.

Original sentence: This clinical study was designed with the purpose of determining the effects of **AB-123** on patients with type 2 diabetes who have coronary artery disease, which is known to place patients at high risk of cardiovascular events. Since **AB-123** was found to reduce the probability of cardiovascular events in animal models, in the present study, it was decided to assess what the effects might be in humans. [67 words]

Revised sentence: The purpose of this clinical study was to determine the **effects** of AB-123 on **patients** with type 2 diabetes who had coronary artery disease. Such **patients** are at high risk of cardiovascular **events**. AB-123 reduced the risk of such **events** in animal models. The present study was designed to determine those **effects** in humans. [54 words]

Refined sentence: Patients with type 2 diabetes and coronary artery disease are at high risk of cardiovascular **events**. Because AB-123 reduces the risk of such **events** in animals, we sought to determine whether it reduces the **risk** in humans. [37 words]

> **Commentary ▶** The revised and refined sentences use different echo words, but both use them effectively. The refined sentence has 37 words and is 55% shorter than the original, which has 67 words. The first and last sentences of the original and revised example both give the purpose of the study. The refined sentence eliminates the duplication.

Chapter 5

Advice for Publishing in English-Language Journals

第 5 章　英文雑誌への投稿時のアドバイス

英文雑誌に投稿する際のキーポイントを具体的にアドバイスする。査読者への返信の仕方などをきめ細かくアドバイス。初心者はもちろん経験豊富な方にも自身のスキルを再確認する上で参考にしてほしい。

Chapter 5

1. Advice for Preparing Scientific Articles
科学論文を作成する際のアドバイス

Tom Lang

■ General Advice

The four questions you need answer are: 1) Why did you start? 2) What did you do? 3) What did you find? and 4) What does it mean? Answer all the questions, first in the abstract and then in the four corresponding parts of the article: Introduction, Methods, Results, and Discussion.

■ Advice for Writing Titles

To write a title, start by identifying the most important parts of your research. Remember SPICED T:

Setting	the setting or location where the study took place
Patients	the diagnosis or characteristics
Intervention	the treatment or exposure
Comparator	the control group or alternative treatment
Endpoint	the outcome of interest
Design	the study design
Time	the date or time period of interest (not always necessary)

The original title has only three of the seven parts:

A Randomized Trial of Low-Air-Loss Beds for Treatment of Pressure Ulcers

The title with all of the SPICED parts."Nursing home"identifies both the location and patients of the study:

Low-Air-Loss Beds vs. Foam Mattresses for Treating Pressure Ulcers in Nursing Home Patients: A Randomized Trial

The revised title is 110 characters, but many journals limit titles to 80 characters. In that case, remove the least-important parts until you meet the limit:

Low-Air-Loss Beds vs. Foam Mattresses for Treating Pressure Ulcers ~~in Nursing Home Patients~~: A Randomized Trial

Removing the reference to patients reduces the title to 86 characters and spaces:

Low-Air-Loss Beds vs. Foam Mattresses for Treating Pressure Ulcers ~~in Nursing Home Patients: A Randomized Trial~~

Finally, removing the reference to patients and the study design is 66 characters and spaces:

Low-Air-Loss Beds vs. Foam Mattresses for Treating Pressure Ulcers

■ Advice for Writing Introductions

Write a four-part introduction consisting of 1) a **background statement** that describes the context of the problem and the research, 2) a **problem statement** that identifies the problem studied and why it is important, 3) an **action statement** that tells what was done to study or solve the problem, and 4) a **forecasting statement** that tell readers what they will find if they continue to read the article.

Consider this original introduction: "Recently, the legislature required the Department of Health to set a minimum nurse-to-patient ratio in acute-care hospitals. We reviewed all studies published between 1980 and 2003 on the effects of some measure of nurse staffing on patient, employee, and hospital outcomes. Thus, we looked for studies that varied the total number of nursing hours or the total number of hours worked by registered nurses on medical-surgical units. Common endpoints included nurse turnover, adverse consequences (eg, pneumonia), and in-hospital mortality. Our results were sent to the State Department of Health and can found in their report to the legislature. We summarize the results here."

Now consider this revised introduction: "**[Background statement]** Cost-containment efforts in recent years have had major consequences for hospitals. Of concern is whether the increased acuity of patients, the increased caregiver workload, and the declining levels of training among patient care personnel have reduced the quality of hospital care. **[Problem statement]** In response, the legislature required the Department of Health to set a minimum nurse-patient ratio in acute-care hospitals. **[Action statement]** We assessed the evidence that might support setting a specific ratio. **[Forecasting statement]** Here, we present the results of a systematic review on the effects of nurse staffing levels on patient, nurse employee, and hospital outcomes in acute-care hospitals. We found little support for setting a specific minimum nurse-patient ratio, especially without also adjusting for case mix and skill mix. "

The original introduction does not include the background or problem statements, which is why it is so difficult to understand.

■ Advice for Writing Results

Lots of numerical results, such as means and standard deviations, *P* values, and confidence intervals, are difficult to read, so put most of them in tables or graphs, not in the text. When citing tables or figures, don't say "The results of the treatment are given in Table 3" say "The treatment shortened time to recovery (Table 3)." In other words, state the meaning of the table and refer readers to it for the supporting data.

In figure captions, avoid saying obvious things, such as "A radiograph of the fracture." Most readers already know what a radiograph looks like. Instead, identify the important parts of the image: "The right femur of a 9-year-old boy fractured when a door was shut on it."

■ Advice for Writing Discussion Sections

Write a seven-part discussion:

Summarize your research and its main findings in a paragraph or two

Interpret the results; tell why you think you did or did not get the results you got

Compare your results with those of others; review the literature and explain why your results are or are not similar

Generalize your results to other patients or circumstances

Speculate about the implications of your research

Critique your research; describe its strengths and limitations

Itemize your conclusions to help you be specific about what your study contributes to the field

2. Advice for Submitting Manuscripts
論文を投稿する際のアドバイス

Mary Shibuya

There is more to submitting a manuscript to a journal than just uploading files. The points discussed below are among the most important considerations.

■ Follow the journal's instruction for authors

All journal editors want to publish research that is new, valid, important, and well reported. They also have to publish articles of high interest to their readers. Therefore, you need to ***read a journal's instructions for authors*** to learn who its readers are, what topics and kinds of articles it wants to publish, and how you should format your manuscript.

Instructions for authors of medical journals around the world are available through links from the University of Toledo Mulford Health Science Library's website: http://mulford.utoledo.edu/instr/.

■ Confirm that all authors meet the criteria for authorship

Most journals require the criteria for authorship developed by the International Committee of Medical Journal Editors (the ICMJE or the Vancouver Group: http://www.icmje.org/). An author is someone who:

1) Has contributed substantially to the research
2) Has contributed substantially to preparing the article
3) Has approved the final version of the article

4) Has agreed to ensure that questions about the work will be investigated and resolved.

Anyone listed as an author must meet all four criteria, and anyone who meets all four criteria should be listed as an author. Persons who contribute to the research but who do not qualify for authorship should be named in the acknowledgements. Persons who do not contribute at all ("ghost" or "guest" authors) should not be listed as authors.

Ideally, authors will be listed in the order of their contributions to the research. The first author is widely accepted as being the most responsible for the research and therefore should receive the most credit. Sometimes, two or more authors want to share the first-author position. However, most journals do not allow more than two co-first authors.

The corresponding author is just the single point of contact for the journal. In the west, the corresponding author has no special importance, so journals allow only a single corresponding author.

■ Provide a clinical trial registration number

Clinical trials must usually be registered as a condition of publication. Common registration numbers include a ClinicalTrials.gov Identifiers, Digital Object Identifiers, and International Standard Randomized Controlled Trial Numbers.

■ Document your research with the appropriate reporting guidelines

Most clinical journals require that research be reported according to standard guidelines. These guidelines are available without charge from the **Equator Network** (Enhancing the QUAlity and Transparency Of health Research; http://www.equator-network.org/). The most commonly used guidelines are CONSORT for reporting randomized controlled trials, STROBE for reporting observational studies, and PRISMA for reporting systematic reviews and meta-analyses.

■ Format your manuscript as directed by the journal

Formatting requirements vary widely from journal to journal. Some editors immediately reject a paper if the formatting is incorrect. More lenient editors, although they may not reject the paper immediately, know that you didn't follow the instructions and wonder how serious you are in publishing in their journal.

Look for the following requirements:

Word and character limits. Many journals limit the number of characters in the title, the number of words in the abstract and text, and sometimes the number of figures and tables.

File formats and naming conventions. The journal may request that graphics and text files be submitted in a certain format and may specify how files are to be named, such as Yamaguchi Fulltext.doc and Takehara Fig 1.jpg.

References and citations. Follow the journal's citing and reference style exactly. Some journals use superscript citations in the text, whereas others use parentheses or brackets to signify the reference number. Many journals follow the American Medical Association's style for formatting references in the bibliography, but other styles are also used.

■ Be prepared to pay the costs of publishing your article

Many journals assess page charges that need to be paid before publication. Open-access journals usually assess article processing fees (APCs), which can range from a few hundred to a few thousand dollars.

■ Keep your cover letter to the editor short

Your cover letter to the editor should be no longer than one page. Describe the question you studied and summarize the results, explaining why your research is important and why it will interest the journal's readers. The letter often contains standard sentences:

"All authors participated in planning, conducting, or analyzing the research, or in drafting or revising the text for intellectual content and have read and approved the submitted version."

"The manuscript has not yet been copyrighted or published and is not currently being considered for publication in another journal." (You do not need to say whether the manuscript has been rejected by another journal, only that it is not currently being considered for publication by another journal.)

3. Advice for Responding to Reviewers
査読者に対応する際のアドバイス

Edward Barroga and Raoul Breugelmans

Publication is the final stage of research. An important and often misunderstood part of this stage is adequately responding to peer reviewers' comments.

A comprehensive approach for authors to pass peer review and to publish includes: 1) accurately interpreting correspondence from the editor, 2) revising the text appropriately, 3) responding to all reviewers' comments, and 4) resubmitting the revisions and response on time.

However, a **major reason manuscripts are rejected on resubmittal after peer review,** even after a favorable and constructive appraisal, is that authors do not adequately respond to the reviewers' comments. To improve their manuscript acceptance rates, Japanese authors must learn how to understand and respond to reviewers. Here, we describe some key points on how to effectively respond to reviewers.

■ Thank the reviewers.

Peer reviewers are unpaid volunteers who are overworked and underappreciated, and they usually review a manuscript after a hard day's work. Yet, most are genuinely devoted to furthering science and they are doing their best to give you honest opinions about your research. Thank them for their in-depth comments and critical appraisal, even if you do not agree with the comments or even if the reviewers seem overly critical. Express your appreciation for their contributions, but do not overdo it. Also, be polite and professional in your responses.

■ Look at the comments from the reviewers' point of view.

Remember that the only information reviewers have about your research is what you give them. They may have to guess at your meaning, and they may guess wrong. Also, criticism is sometimes not easy to receive. So, before you write your responses, think about them for a few days, after any strong emotions have passed.

■ Respond to every comment, whether it appears to be important or not.

You cannot choose the comments you want or can respond to and leave the rest unanswered. The editor may think that you do not know how to respond or that you do not want to admit that you made serious mistakes in your research. In either case, your credibility as a researcher will be questioned, which is not to your advantage. In fact, not responding to some comments may mean having your paper rejected.

Carefully analyze each comment to be sure you understand it. Then, provide a careful, complete, and professional response to each one. Many times, reviewers ask for clarification. Thus, it is crucial to provide a clear explanation with sufficient background, detail, and perhaps references about what you did and why. Your response does not have to be long. If you agree with the reviewer, just write "We agree with the reviewer and have made the change." If you do not agree with the reviewer—and you should feel free to—explain why you disagree and chose not to make the requested change.

A common unhelpful response is, "We have made the changes in the text" with no further explanation in your letter. This response irritates reviewers and journal editors; they want to read your changes in your response letter and not have to find the changes in the manuscript. So, you should copy all the substantive changes in the manuscript and place them in your response to the comments. Indicate the page and paragraph (and line numbers, if the journal requires them) in which the changes appear in the manuscript.

■ Clearly mark all revisions in the manuscript so they can be found and read easily.

In the manuscript, indicate all your changes by a) underlining, b) using bold face, c) using a different font color, d) highlighting, or e) using the tracking mode following the journal requirements.

■ Have your co-authors and, if possible, a professional editor re-check and re-edit the revised manuscript and response letter.

All authors need to be involved in responding to the reviewers' comments and in approving the revised manuscript. Ideally, the editor will be experienced and will have some knowledge of your specialty. If possible, request that the editor who edited the presubmittal manuscript be the one to review the responses and revisions.

■ Review all revised files before resubmittal.

Give yourself time to revise the manuscript and to respond to the reviewers; do not wait until the last minute. Make sure the changes are clearly marked in the manuscript and are consistent with those in the response letter. Label all files according to the resubmittal instructions.

■ Conclusions

Peer review is as old as the scientific journal. However, it does not always work as hoped. Agreement among peer reviewers on the same manuscript is often not much better than chance, and peer review has not prevented the publication of poor or even fraudulent research. At the same time, most authors agree that peer review *does* improve scientific communications, and almost all agree that peer review has improved the quality of their own papers.

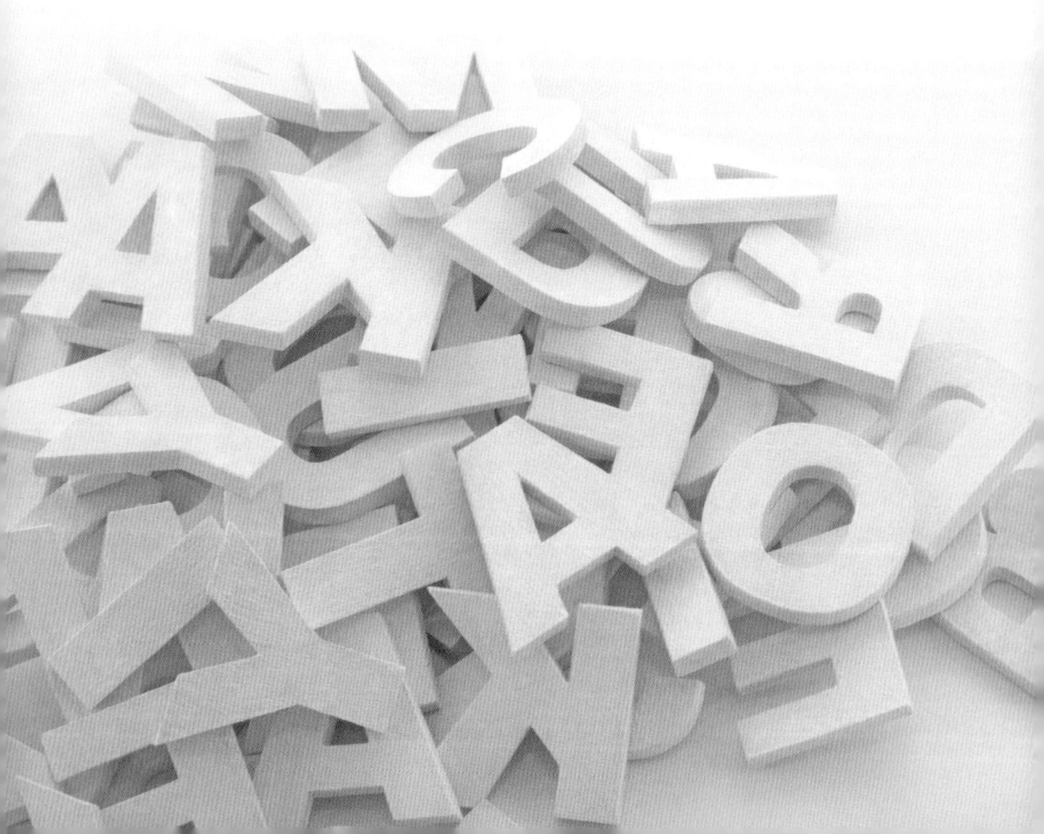

References 文献

1. American Medical Association. *AMA Manual of Style: A Guide for Authors and Editors, 10th Edition*. New York: Oxford University Press, 2007.

2. Byrne DW. *Publishing Your Medical Research, 2nd edition*. Alphen aan den Rijn, The Netherlands: Wolters Kluwer, 2017.

3. Council of Science Editors. *Scientific Style and Format: The CSE Manual for Authors, Editors, and Publishers, 8th edition*. Chicago: University of Chicago Press, 2006.

4. Gastel B, Day RA. *How to Write and Publish a Scientific Paper, 8th edition*. Santa Barbara, CA: ABC-CLIO, 2016.

5. Gopen, George D. *The Common Sense of Writing: Teaching Writing from the Reader's Perspective*, 1990.

6. Heinemann M. *How NOT to Write a Medical Paper: A Practical Guide*. Delhi: Thieme Medical and Scientific Publishers, 2016.

7. Lang T. Choosing and Communicating with Journals. *J Pub Health Emerg*. 2018. doi: 10.21037/jphe.2018.01.02

8. Lang T. *How to Write, Publish, and Present in the Health Sciences: A Guide for Clinicians and Laboratory Researchers*. Philadelphia: American College of Physicians, 2010. **Japanese translation**, 2011.

9. Lang T. Writing a better research article. *J Pub Health Emerg*. 2017. doi: 10.21037/jphe.2017.11.06

10. Williams JM. *Style: Ten Lessons in Clarity and Grace. Glenview, Illinois*: Scott, Foresman, & Co., 1988.

11. Zinsser W. *On Writing Well*. New York: Harper Collins; 2006. ISBN 978-0-06-089154-1.

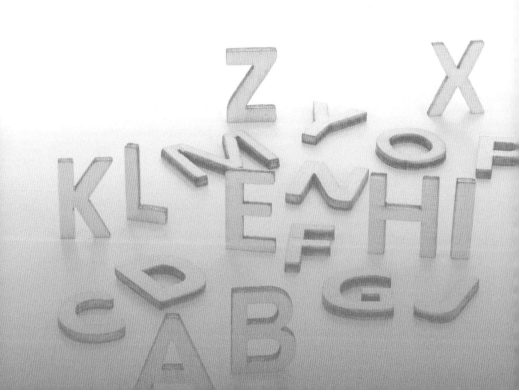

Afterword あとがき

After the big earthquake in northeastern Japan in 2011, many Japanese scientists lost their research, sometimes a lifetime of work. I wanted to do something to help, but what could I do? I didn't even live in Japan. But I realized that I could do one small thing; I could focus on assisting Japanese researchers with their English medical writing. It would not help those researchers immediately, but maybe in the future they would rebuild their research, and then they could communicate that research more effectively in English. After that, I began to work more on medical writing, and to develop the 3Cs method. Then a friend said, "You should write a book." I didn't know anything about writing a book, but my mentor and expert medical writer Tom Lang agreed to be my co-author, my friends and colleagues Raoul Breugelmans, Edward Barroga, and Mary Shibuya agreed to contribute, and the wonderful team at Life Science Publishing encouraged me and helped to shape the book. Their support, cooperation, and encouragement brought this book into reality. Any errors are mine alone.

Lee Seaman

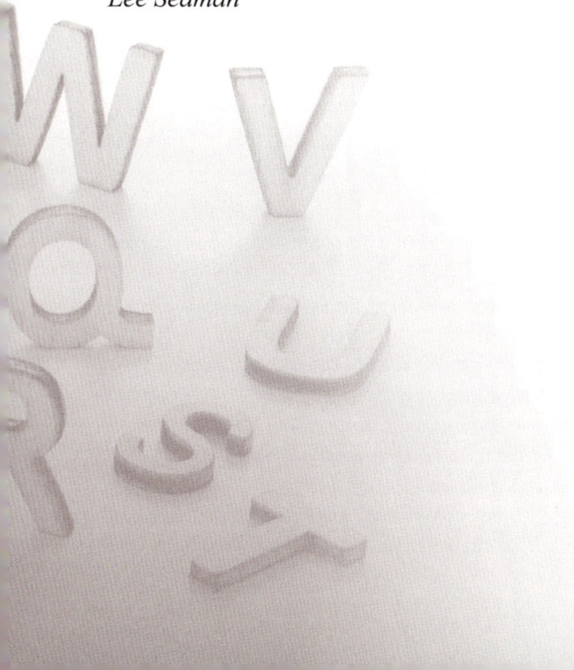

About the Authors and Contributors

執筆者・協力者

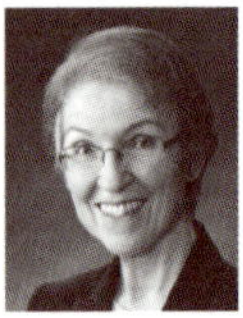

Lee Seaman

Lee Seaman was born and raised in rural Eastern Oregon, USA. She did undergraduate work in chemistry and biology at Oregon State University and studied for a year at the International Division of Waseda University. After graduation, she returned to Japan to teach English, pursue further Japanese language study, and begin translating technical documents, such as drug patents and clinical study reports from Japanese to English. After 10 years in Japan, Lee returned to the USA. In 2000 she founded Seaman Medical, Inc., and began to assist Japanese authors who needed to present their research in English to the international medical community. Clearly, "literal translation" was not enough; to establish clear communication, the principles of medical writing were required. However, most books and presentations were designed for writers with native or near-native proficiency in English, leaving many Japanese authors struggling to prepare English-language documents. Lee has been working since 2010 to fill that gap. She works from her office in Bellingham, Washington, and makes twice-yearly trips to Japan to attend Japanese medical and pharmaceutical conferences and to present workshops on English medical writing for Japanese native speakers who want to gain confidence in their English writing skills.

For help with translation, editing, and medical writing, or to schedule a workshop or online training in 3Cs English, contact:

Lee Seaman, President
Seaman Medical, Inc.
lseaman@seamanmedical.com
www.seamanmedical.com

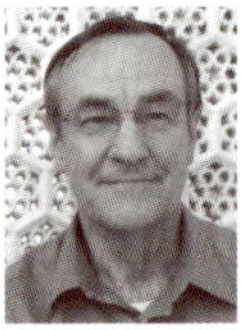

Tom Lang, MA

Tom Lang, MA, has been a medical-technical writer-editor since 1975. Now an international consultant and educator in medical and professional communications, he was Manager of Medical Editing Services at the Cleveland Clinic for many years and worked at the New England Cochrane and Evidence-Based Practice Centers as a senior medical writer-editor. He has taught regularly in Japan and throughout Asia for more than 20 years. His books, *How to Report Statistics in Medicine* and *How to Write, Publish, and Present in the Health Sciences*, are standard references in evidence-based medicine and medical writing. Both books have been translated into Japanese. He was part of the original CONSORT and PRISMA groups, which developed guidelines for reporting randomized trials and systematic reviews, respectively. He has taught on the University of Chicago's Medical Writing Program since its beginning in 1999 and has received teaching awards from the American Statistical Association, the

University of Chicago, and the American Medical Writers Association. A Past President of the Council of Science Editors, he is also the current Financial Officer of the World Association of Medical Editors. His master's degree in Communications Management is from the Annenberg School for Communications at the University of Southern California.

For help with preparing scientific publications and conference communications and for training in medical writing and editing, understanding statistics, and research documentation, contact:

Tom Lang, Principal
Tom Lang Communications and Training International
tomlangcom@aol.com
www.tomlangcommunications.com

Contributors

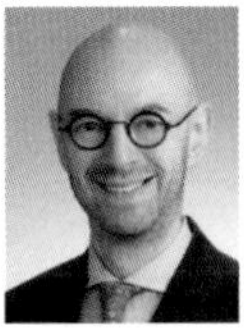

Raoul Breugelmans

Raoul Breugelmans is originally from Antwerp, Belgium. He completed undergraduate studies in linguistics at the University of Oregon, USA, including a year on an exchange program at the International Division of Waseda University, Japan. He received a master's degree (1991) and completed the doctoral course (ABD, 1994) in Japanese philology at Meiji University, Japan. Since 2002 he has been a full-time faculty member of Tokyo Medical University, where he has been involved in biomedical editing, teaching of English for medical purposes, medical education, and development and administration of information and communication technology systems. He currently heads the Department of English. He serves as Director of the Japan Society for Medical English Education, Director of the Japanese Society of Travel Medicine, and Councilor of the Japan Society for Medical Education. He has assisted hundreds of Japanese researchers in publishing their work in the international literature and lectures throughout Japan on various aspects of international medical communications.

Contact information:

Raoul Breugelmans
rpb@tokyo-med.ac.jp

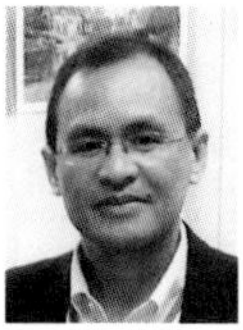

Edward Barroga, PhD

Edward Barroga holds a PhD in Veterinary Surgery/Oncology (differentiation therapy of osteosarcoma) from Hokkaido University, Japan, and a DVM (Internal Medicine/Pathology) from the University of the Philippines. He has over 25 years of experience as an academician, department chairman, researcher, author, and reviewer. Dr. Barroga is a professor of academic writing at St. Luke's International University (SLIU) in Tokyo. He was previously an associate professor of medical education and of medical communications at Tokyo Medical University (TMU). He has extensive experience in medical/academic writing, editing, and publishing. This involves daily manuscript editing and consultations with Japanese medical doctors and professionals as biomedical and senior medical editor for over 15 years. He also co-developed the academic writing desk program of SLIU. Dr. Barroga was a DuPont outstanding young scientist awardee and an international advisory board member of European Science Editing. He is well published in biomedicine and in medical editing, writing, and publishing.

Contact information:

Edward Barroga, PhD
barrogas@gmail.com
http://orcid.org/0000-0002-8920-2607

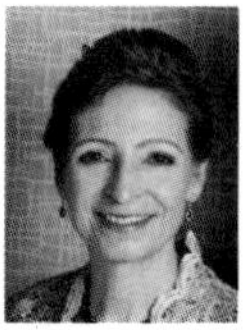

Mary Shibuya

Mary Shibuya is an American medical editor-writer with a background in chemistry and allergy research at the Mayo Clinic in Rochester, MN, who has lived in Japan since 1983. For 23 years she was the language editor of *Internal Medicine*, a journal published by the Japanese Society of Internal Medicine. In addition to preparing and editing research articles for publication in international journals, she conducts interviews at medical and scientific congresses as a representative of the scientific press and transcribes and summarizes conference proceedings. She gives presentations on medical writing in English at Japanese pharmaceutical companies and medical conferences, lectures on scientific writing in English at Gunma University Graduate School of Medicine, and constantly strives to encourage Japanese doctors and researchers to publish in English-language, peer-reviewed journals.

Contact information:

Mary Shibuya
mary77gauerke81sto@gmail.com
http://mary-shibuya.strikingly.com

造　本：廣瀬亮平（廣瀬デザイン室）
編　集：毛利公子
山口ちとせ

世界に通じるメディカルライティング
ネイティブライターが伝授する3Cs English
International Medical Writing: English for a Global Audience

2019年4月25日 初版第1刷発行

著　者：Lee Seaman, Tom Lang

発行人：須永光美
発行所：ライフサイエンス出版株式会社
〒105-0014 東京都港区芝 3-5-2
代表　TEL.03-6275-1522
書籍編集部　TEL.03-6275-1524　FAX.03-6275-1527
会社 HP http://www.lifescience.co.jp/

印刷・製本：三報社印刷株式会社

Printed in Japan
ISBN 978-4-89775-388-1 C3047